Pops

by Charlotte Josephine

Produced in a co-production with
Jake Orr Productions, HighTide and Live Theatre.

Pops was first performed at Assembly Roxy at the
Edinburgh Festival Fringe on 2nd August 2019

CAST
Sophie Melville – Daughter
Nigel Barrett – Father

CREATIVES
Charlotte Josephine – Writer
Ali Pidsley – Director
Bethany Wells – Designer
Kieran Lucas – Sound Designer
Anna Reddyhoff – Lighting Designer
Jennifer Jackson – Movement Director
Live Theatre and HighTide – Dramaturgy
Jake Orr – Producer
Gareth Edwards – Production Manager
Rose Hockaday – Stage Manager
Chloé Nelkin Consulting – PR

CAST

Sophie Melville – Daughter

Sophie trained at Royal Welsh College of Music and Drama.

Theatre credits include: *Wolfie* (Theatre503); *Blue* (Chapter Theatre); *Close Quarters* (Sheffield Crucible); *Pops* (Young Vic); *No One Will Tell Me How to Start a Revolution* (Hampstead Theatre); *The Divide* and *Pagans* (Old Vic); *Low Level Panic* (Orange Tree Theatre); *2066* (Almeida Theatre); *Blackbird* (The Other Room Theatre, Winner: Best Female Performance, Wales Theatre Awards); *Insignificance* (Theatr Clwyd); *Iphigenia in Splott* (National Theatre, Theater 59E59 NYC, The Sherman, Edinburgh Fringe Festival and International Tour, Winner: The Stage Award for Acting Excellence and Best Female Performance, Wales Theatre Award. Evening Standard Award nomination for Best Actress, Drama Desk Award nomination for Outstanding Solo Performance); *Romeo and Juliet* (The Sherman Theatre); *Under Milk Wood* (Theatr Clwyd Cymru); *The Shape of Things*; *'Tis a Pity She's a Whore*; *See How They Run* (Theatre by the Lake); *Romeo and Juliet* (The Sam Wanamaker Festival).

Television credits include: *The Left Behind, The Missing 2* (BBC).

Nigel Barrett – Father

Theatre credits include: *The Show In Which Hopefully Nothing Happens* (Unicorn Theatre); *Mysteries* (Royal Exchange); *100: Unearthed* (Wildworks); *Party Skills for the End of the World* (Manchester International Festival and Shoreditch Town Hall); *Kingdom Come* (Royal Shakespeare Company); *margate/dreamland* (Shoreditch Town Hall); *Blasted* (Barrel Organ / STYX); *Baddies the Musical* (Unicorn Theatre); *The Eye Test* (National Theatre); *Everyone* (Chris Goode and Co); *The Iphigenia Quartet* (The Gate); *Cyrano de Bergerac* (Northern Stage); *Praxis Makes Perfect* (National Theatre Wales / Berlin Festspiele); *Mad Man* (Theatre Royal Plymouth); *There Has Possibly Been an Incident* (Royal Exchange); *Get Stuff Break Free* (National Theatre); *The Passion* (National Theatre Wales / Wildworks); *Pericles (Regent's Park)* and *Richard III – An Arab Tragedy (Royal Shakespeare Company)*.

Film and Television credits include: *Doctors* (BBC); *Cycles* (Toynbee Film); *The Gospel of Us, The Boat, Hello You, Casualty, Meet the Piltdowns, Hairy Eyeball, Dawson's Creek Special, The Mysteries, Deadline, The Lens, Sexual Healing, England My England*. Nigel is a member of the shunt collective and works extensively with Louise Mari.

www.nigelandlouise.com.

CREATIVE TEAM

Charlotte Josephine – Writer

Charlotte Josephine is an award-winning playwright represented by The Agency, and actor represented by Hatton McEwan Penford. In 2012 *Bitch Boxer* won the Soho Theatre Young Writers Award, the Old Vic New Voices Edinburgh Season 2012, the Clonmel Junction Best Theatre Award 2013, the Holden Street Theatre's Award 2013 and the Adelaide Fringe Award 2014.

'Sweat-slicked and tough, yet sweet and gifted with terrific timing' *The Times*
'A pumped up underdog with a big heart' *The Independent*

In 2016 *Blush* won The Stage Edinburgh Award.
'It's riveting' *The Times*
'Vital theatre' *The Stage*
'Powerful and important theatre' *The Telegraph*

In 2017 Charlotte won the inaugural BBC Screenplay First Award, and was named on the BBC New Talent Hotlist. Charlotte is currently under commission at Boundless Theatre, Audible, Theatre Centre and BBC Films.

Ali Pidsley – Director

Ali is a Director & Theatre-Maker from Yorkshire. He is a founding member of award-winning theatre collective Barrel Organ, for whom he directed their award-winning debut production *NOTHING*. Ali is an Alumni Artist of the Gate Theatre and is a Leverhulme Arts Scholar. In 2014 he was the recipient of the Buzz Goodbody Award for Directing.

For Barrel Organ: *Some People Talk About Violence* & *NOTHING* (Camden People's Theatre, Edinburgh Festival Fringe & UK Tour).

Other theatre directing includes: *A Girl in School Uniform (Walks Into a Bar)* (Leeds Playhouse & New Diorama Theatre); *Blasted* (Styx Tottenham, RIFT Theatre); *Left Luggage* (The Space, Kimbo Theatre) and *Danielle* (Slingshot Manchester).

As Assistant/ Associate Director, Ali has worked with the National Theatre, Headlong, Chichester Festival Theatre, Royal Exchange & Manchester International Festival, Leeds Playhouse & Forced Entertainment.

Ali is proud to work as a selector for the National Student Drama Festival.

Bethany Wells – Designer

Bethany trained in architecture, she is a performance designer working across dance, theatre and installation, with a particular interest in site-specific and devised performance. Bethany sees all design as a form of activism, and is interested in exploring what can be achieved politically and socially by the collective live experience of performance. Bethany is an Associate Artist with Middle Child, Hull.

Recent work includes: *Thank You Very Much*, Claire Cunningham, MIF, *All That Lives*, Grief Series, Leeds International Festival, *Us Against Whatever*, Middle Child, *The War of The Worlds*, Rhum + Clay, *Rallying Cry*, Battersea Arts Centre, *Busking It*, High Tide, *DISTANCE*, Park Theatre, *A New And Better You*, Yard Theatre, *TRUST*, Gate Theatre, *Party Skills for the End of the World*, Nigel Barrett and Louise Mari, MIF, *The Department of Distractions*, Third Angel, *All We Ever Wanted Was Everything*, Middle Child.

Work in development includes: *STORM* and *Search Party*.

An ongoing project, *WARMTH*, is a wood-fired mobile sauna and performance space, commissioned by Compass Live Art.

Winner, BEST SET DESIGN for Distance, Park Theatre, OffWestEnd Awards [2018]

www.bethanywells.com

Kieran Lucas – Sound Designer

Kieran is a sound designer and theatre-maker and also helps to run Streatham Space Project in South London.

Sound & composition credits include: *Orlando* (Vaults); *Mydidae* (Hope Mill Theatre); *How We Save The World* (Natural History Museum); *The Ex-Boyfriend Yard Sale* (CPT/Progress Festival); *TBCTV* (Somerset House); *Gastronomic* (Norwich Theatre Royal); *Square Go* (Paines Plough Roundabout); *I Wanna Be Yours* (Paines Plough/Tamasha UK Tour); *The Ministry of Memory* (Imperial War Museum North); *The Drill* (BAC/UK Tour); *A Girl In School Uniform (Walks Into A Bar)* (New Diorama) – Off-West End award nominated for Best Sound Design, Theatre & Technology award nominated for Best Sound Design, *The Shadow of the Future* (Imperial War Museum); *Anyone's Guess How We Got Here* (ZOO/UK Tour); *REMOTE* (CPT/UK Tour); *My Name Is Rachel Corrie* (Young Vic); *BIG GUNS* (The Yard); *Under The Skin* (St. Paul's Cathedral); *Some People Talk About Violence* (Summerhall/UK Tour) and *NOTHING* (Summerhall/UK Tour).

Anna Reddyhoff – Lighting Designer

Anna has been working within the entertainment industry for almost 10 years after graduating in 2010. She is thrilled to be working on the creative team on *Pops*.

Previous Lighting Design credits include: *The Re-Birth of Meadow Rain* (Edinburgh Festival 2019); *The Lion, The Witch and The Wardrobe* (Lichfield Garrick Theatre); *Reformation* (The White Bear); *Flinch* (The Old Red Lion); *Emilia* (Vaudeville Theatre) (Associate LD to Zoe Spurr); *Heart The Play* (The Vaults London); *Sara Pascoe: Lads Lads Lads* (Wyndham's Theatre); *Tim Vine: Sunset Milk Idiot* (Hammersmith Apollo); *One Man, Two Guvnors* (Lichfield Garrick); *Once Upon a Mattress* (Lichfield Garrick) and *Rent* (A3 Arena).

Other selected credits include: *Re-Lighter: Transporting Live* (UK Tour – Seabright Productions); Chief Electrician – *Moulin Rouge* (Secret Cinema); Deputy Chief Electrician – *Chitty Chitty Bang Bang* (UK Tour – Music & Lyrics Ltd); Deputy Head of Lighting and Video – *Hairspray* (UK Tour – Mark Goucher Lt).

Jennifer Jackson – Movement Director

Jennifer trained at East 15 and is a movement director and actor. Movement direction includes: *Death of a Salesman*, *Queens of the Coal Age*, *Our Town* (Royal Exchange Theatre); *Parliament Square*, *Philoxenia/The Trick* (Bush Theatre/Royal Exchange Theatre); *Out of Water/ Mayfly* (Orange Tree); *Around the World In 80 Days/ Be My Baby* (Leeds Playhouse); *The Strange Undoing of Prudencia Hart* (New Vic); *Brighton Rock* (Pilot Theatre /The Lowry); *Island Town/ Sticks and Stones/ How to Spot an Alien* (PainesPlough Roundabout); *The Mountaintop* (Young Vic & Tour); *Black Mountain/ How to be a Kid /Out of Love* (Paines Plough & Orange Tree); *Death of a Salesman* (Royal & Derngate); *The Ugly One* (Park Theatre); *Why The Whales Came* (Southbank Centre); *Stone Face* (Finborough Theatre); *Debris* (Southwark Playhouse/Openworks Theatre); *Macbeth* (Passion in Practice/Sam Wanamaker Playhouse); *Silent Planet* (Finborough); *Pericles* (Berwaldhallen); *The Future* (The Yard/Company Three) and *Other-Please Specify*, *Atoms* (Company Three); *Takeover 2017* (Kiln Theatre).

Assistant movement director credits include: *Lungs*, *The Initiate*, *My Teacher's a Troll* (Paines Plough Roundabout 2014). Jennifer is a Leverhulme Arts Scholar, and is currently developing *Thank Heaven For Little Girls* with The egg, The Lowry and The Place.

Jake Orr – Producer

Jake is Producer for Theatre503 and Jake Orr Productions. Before joining Theatre503 Jake was a freelance producer and programmer. In 2009 he founded A Younger Theatre, an organisation that supports and nurtures young people through journalism training. In 2014 Jake co-founded Incoming Festival with New Diorama Theatre, a festival that supports emerging theatre companies. Jake is also co-director of producing company Making Room.

Jake's producing credits include: *Wolfie* (Theatre503); *Cinderella and the Beanstalk* (Theatre503); *Br'er Cotton* (Theatre503, Winner: Best New Play OffWestEnd Awards); *In Event of Moone Disaster* (Theatre503, Winner: Best New Writer The Stage Debut Awards); *No Miracles Here* (The Letter Room at Edinburgh Festival Fringe, Northern Stage, The Lowry and Shoreditch Town Hall); *BLUSH* (Snuff Box Theatre at Edinburgh Fringe Festival, Soho and on Tour, Winner: The Stage Award for Best Performance); *Weald* (Snuff Box Theatre and Finborough Theatre) and *Shelter me* (Circumference and Theatre Delicatessen). He has also produced Dialogue Festival (Ovalhouse).

As co-producer his credits include: *J'Ouvert* (Theatre503); *The Art of Gaman* (Theatre503); *Gutted* (HOME, Manchester and Edinburgh Festival Fringe); *COW* (Edinburgh Festival Fringe) and *Sticking* (National Tour).

As Associate Producer his credits include: *Lists for the End of the World* (Edinburgh Festival Fringe); *The Bombing of the Grand Hotel* (Cockpit Theatre and Tour); *Mouse Plague* (Edinburgh Festival Fringe, BAC and Tour) and *The Eradication of Schizophrenia in Western Lapland* (Edinburgh Festival Fringe, BAC and Tour). Jake was nominated for Best Producer in the 2014 OffWestEnd Awards.

Gareth Edwards – Production Manager

Gareth trained at Rose Bruford College in Theatre Design. Since graduating, he has worked exclusively as a Production Manager. Recent Credits includes: *Frankenstein* (National Tour); *The Rink*, *The Fall* and *DNA* (Southwark Playhouse); *Tiny Dynamite* (The Old Red Lion); *A Christmas Tale* (Kenton Theatre); *The Sound and The Fury* (Pleasance Theatre).

Musical Theatre includes: *The War of the Worlds* (The Dominion Theatre, London); *Carrie* (Southwark Playhouse); *The Sound of Music* (UK Tour); *The Glenn Miller Story* (UK Tour); *Blood Brothers*

(UK Tour); *Joseph* (UK Tour); *Imaginary* (The Other Palace, London); *Love's Labour's Lost* (Hackney Empire, London); *Dancing in the Streets* (UK Tour); *HONK* (UK Tour); *Billy The Kid* (The Curve, Leicester); *Sunday in the Park* (The Other Palace, London); *Yank* (Charing Cross Theatre, London); *Evita* (Dominion Theatre & UK Tour) and Imaginary (The Other Palace).

Plays include: *Rehearsal for Murder* (UK Tour); *Before The Party* (UK Tour); *Twelve Angry Men* (UK Tour); *Shawshank Redemption* (UK Tour); *The Small Hand* (UK Tour); *And Then There Were None* (UK Tour); *The Common Pursuit* (Menier Chocolate Factory); *Yerma* (Battersea Arts Center) and *Triptych* (Southwark Playhouse).

Pantomime includes: *Aladdin* (Regent Theatre, Stoke on Trent); *Beauty and The Beast* (Theatre Royal, Nottingham); (New Theatre Cardiff); *Jack & the Beanstalk* (Theatre Royal, Nottingham) and *Aladdin* (His Majesty's Theatre, Aberdeen).

Opera and Ballet credits include: *Threepenny Opera* (Shoreditch Town Hall, London); *Too Hot to Handel* (UK Tour); *A Little Princess* (Peacock Theatre, London); *Pelleas & Melisande* (Irish Tour) and *Alcina* (Irish Tour).

International credits include: *Jesus Christ Superstar* (UK / German Tour); *Testing the Echo* (The Hague); *Rum & Vodka* (Sao Paulo); *The Good Thief* (Sao Paulo); *Thriller Live* (Europe and World Tour) and *Pendragon* (Japanese Tour).

Rose Hockaday – Stage Manager

Rose graduated from Rose Bruford College in 2014 with a degree in Lighting Design, and has since been working as a Freelance Lighting Technician & Stage Manager in London.

Theatre credits include: *The Ex-Boyfriend Yard Sale* (Camden Peoples Theatre); *Wolfie, Art of Gaman* (Theatre 503); *You Only Live Forever, In Tents and Purposes* (Viscera Theatre); *Timmy; Glitter Punch; Sophie, Ben and Other Problems; The Festival of Spanish Theatre; How To Survive A Post-Truth Apocalypse; They Built It. No One Came, and Jericho Creek* (Fledgling Theatre); *A View From Islington North* (Out of Joint) and *The Angry Brigade* (Paines Plough).

Film credits include: *Heaven Knows, Visitors, Ignite, Pomegranate, Wandering Eyes* and *Versions of Us*. As well as music videos *Phase Me Out*, When *You're Gone*, and *Saint* for artist VÉRITÉ.

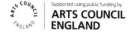 Supported using public funding by
ARTS COUNCIL
ENGLAND

The *Pops* team would like to thank; Young Vic, Ovalhouse, Imogen Knight, Sean Campion and Holly Aston for their time and support during the research and development phases of *Pops*. Thank you to Allan Wilson, Michael Smiley, the Live Theatre and HighTide teams including Joe Douglas and Steven Atkinson for their support.

Jake Orr Productions (JOP) was founded in 2019 as a production company producing new plays, theatre and work across the UK, led by producer Jake Orr. JOP's mission is to inspire and change society, one play at a time.

JOP's inaugural production is *Pops* by Charlotte Josephine. Future JOP plays are in research and development with writers and artists.

JOP would like to thank Jack Lynch, Michelle Barnette, Liam McLaughlin and Desara Bosnja for their support and encouragement.

www.jakeorr.co.uk
@JakeOrrProd
facebook.com/JakeOrrProd

H|GH T|DE

NEW THEATRE FOR
ADVENTUROUS PEOPLE

HighTide is a theatre company and charity based in East Anglia that has an unparalleled twelve-year history of successfully launching the careers of emerging British playwrights.

Our alumni speak for themselves: Luke Barnes, Adam Brace, Tallulah Brown, E V Crowe, Elinor Cook, Rob Drummond, Thomas Eccleshare, Theresa Ikoko, Branden Jacobs-Jenkins, Eve Leigh, Anders Lustgarten, Joel Horwood, Ella Hickson, Harry Melling, Nessah Muthy, Vinay Patel, Nick Payne, Phil Porter, Beth Steel, Al Smith, Sam Steiner, Molly Taylor, Jack Thorne and Frances Ya-Chu Cowhig.

We have staged productions with the highest quality theatres across the UK, from the Traverse in Edinburgh, to the Royal Exchange in Manchester, Theatre Royal Bath and the National Theatre in London. We discover new talent, provide creative development opportunities for playwrights and other creatives, and stage high quality theatre productions both in our region and nationally through our festivals and touring.

We enable new and underrepresented playwrights to express their visions of contemporary politics and society, demonstrate their creative potential and therein showcase the future of theatre.

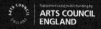

ARTS COUNCIL ENGLAND
Supported using public funding by

LANSONS
Advice Ideas Results

BackstageTrust

H|GH T|DE

2019
TWELVE YEARS OF
SHAPING THE MAINSTREAM

Our twelfth season under Artistic Director Steven Atkinson, began in February 2019 with Eve Leigh's **The Trick**, directed by Roy Alexander Weise in a HighTide and Loose Tongue co-production. **The Trick** premiered at the Bush Theatre before embarking on an national tour.

In April, **Mouthpiece** by Kieran Hurley, presented by Traverse Theatre in association with HighTide transfered to Soho Theatre after a successful run at Traverse Theatre in December 2018. It will return to Edinburgh in August as part of the Traverse's Edinburgh Festival Fringe 2019 season.

Rust by Kenny Emson, directed by Eleanor Rhode, will be presented in a HighTide and Bush Theatre co-production in June 2019 at the Bush Theatre. **Rust** will transfer to the Edinburgh Festival Fringe before running at HighTide Festival in September 2019.

HighTide, in partnership with Assembly Roxy, launch **Disruption: The Future of New Theatre** as part of the Edinburgh Festival Fringe 2019. **Disruption** will present a curated programme of provocative and contemporary new theatre. Alongside **Rust**, HighTide will co-produce a further four productions: **Pops** by Charlotte Josephine, **Collapsible** by Margaret Perry, **Since U Been Gone** by Teddy Lamb & **Pink Lemonade** by Mia Johnson.

Former HighTide First Commissions Writer Sophie Ellerby will premiere **LIT** in September 2019, directed by Stef O'Driscoll in a HighTide and Nottingham Playhouse co-production. **LIT** will debut at the HighTide Festival before transferring to Nottingham Playhouse.

Finally, HighTide are partnering with **BBC Radio 3** and **BBC Arts** on two new radio plays by HighTide alumni writers Tallulah Brown and Vinay Patel. These plays will be presented at HighTide Festival in 2019 with a live recording to be broadcast later this year.

For full details, visit hightide.org.uk

HIGH TIDE

HIGHTIDE THEATRE

24a St John Street, London, EC1M 4AY
0207 566 9765 - hello@hightide.org.uk - hightide.org.uk

HighTide Company

Artistic Director Steven Atkinson
Artistic Director Designate Suba Das
Executive Producer Francesca Clark
Executive Producer (Maternity Cover) Rowan Rutter
Producer Robyn Keynes
Assistant Producer Holly White
Festival Producer, Aldeburgh Elizabeth Downie
Marketing and Communications Officer Kathleen Smith

Associate Writers:

Taj Atwal, William Drew, Sonia Jalaly, James McDermott, Yolanda Mercy

Board

Steven Atkinson; Tim Clark (Chair); Nancy Durrant; Sue Emmas; Liz Fosbury; Jon Gilchrist; Diana Hiddleston; Priscilla John; Clare Parsons; Vinay Patel; John Rodgers; Leah Schmidt; Graham White (Deputy Chair)

Festival Board, Aldeburgh

Tallulah Brown; Andrew Clarke; Tim Clark (HighTide chair); Heather Newill; Ruth Proctor; Jenni Wake-Walker; Caroline Wiseman

Patrons

Stephen Daldry CBE; Sir Richard Eyre CBE; Sally Greene OBE; Sir David Hare; Sir Nicholas Hytner; Sam Mendes CBE; Juliet Stevenson CBE.

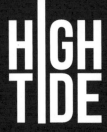

HIGH TIDE

BE A FRIEND OF THE FESTIVAL

"There are very talented young playwrights in the UK and if they are lucky they will find their way to HighTide Theatre. I hope you will join me in supporting this remarkable and modest organisation. With your help HighTide can play an even more major role in the promoting of new writing in the UK."
Lady Susie Sainsbury, Backstage Trust

Our Friends are an important part of HighTide. Our benefits include:
- An invite to the Festival programme launch party in Aldeburgh
- An invite to the Artists and Friends Brunch during the Festival
- Dedicated ticket booking service and access to house seats for sold out events

From as little as £10 a month, your contribution will support the Festival in providing:
- Performance tickets to local school children
- Workshops on performance and writing
- The Summer Connect club in Aldeburgh for the next generation of playwrights

All of which we can provide at no cost to local young people, thanks to the generosity of our Friends.

Be a Friend for as little as £10 per month, or become a Best Friend for as little as £25 per month.

To make a one-off contribution, please call our offices on 01728 687110 quoting `Friends of the Festival', or email **rowan@hightide.org.uk**.

We are thankful to all of our supporters, without whom our work simply would not take place.

HighTide Theatre is a National Portfolio Organisation of the Arts Council England

live theatre

Live Theatre is dedicated to developing and producing new plays, by discovering, nurturing and championing new talent. It is the only English new writing theatre, outside London, to do this.

For almost 50 years, Live Theatre has been creating compelling, award-winning plays that speak to the people of the North East, with universal truths that appeal to a broad, national and international audience.

Located on Newcastle upon Tyne's Quayside, Live Theatre is based in a carefully restored complex of five Grade II listed buildings, combining state-of-the-art facilities in a unique historical setting with a flexible and welcoming theatre space, studio, rehearsal room and writers' rooms. Live Theatre draws on a broad portfolio of income streams and is recognised as a national leader in developing new strategies for increasing income and assets to support its work.

Live Theatre's Best Friends

Anthony Atkinson, Jim Beirne, Michael & Pat Brown, Paul Callaghan & Dorothy Braithwaite, George Caulkin, Michael & Susan Chaplin, Sue & Simon Clugson, Christine Elton, David & Gitta Faulkner, Chris Foy, Robson Green, Lee Hall, Brenna Hobson, John Josephs, Graham Maddick, Madelaine Newton, Dianne, Ian & Christine Shepherdson, Shelagh Stephenson, Sting, Alan Tailford, Graeme & Aly Thompson, Paul & Julie Tomlinson, Alison Walton, Lucy Winskell, and others that choose to remain anonymous.

Live Theatre, Broad Chare, Quayside, Newcastle, NE1 3DQ

For more information see www.live.org.uk

Twitter & Facebook: @LiveTheatre
Instagram @LiveTheatreNewcastle

Live Theatre is the trading name of North East Theatre Trust, a registered charity number 513771

John Ellerman Foundation

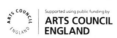

Live Theatre Staff

Chief Executive Jim Beirne
PA to CEO and Finance Assistant Clare Overton

Customer Services
Customer Service Team Leader Nichola Ivey
Duty Manager Grace Blamire
Duty Manager Michael Davies
Duty Manager Lewis Jobson
Duty Manager Ben Young

Creative Programme
Artistic Director Joe Douglas
Emeritus Artistic Director Max Roberts
Creative Producer Graeme Thompson
Creative Programme Administrator John Dawson
Creative Associate Programming Anna Ryder

Children and Young People
Children and Young People's Programme Leader Helen Green
Senior Creative Associate CYP Paul James
Creative Associate CYP Toni McElhatton (maternity leave)
Creative Associate CYP (Maternity Cover) Becky Morris
Creative Lead Live Tales Ross Wylie
Live Tales Volunteer Coordinator Izzie Hutchinson

Technical & Production
Production Manager Drummond Orr
Technical & Digital Manager Dave Flynn
Technician Craig Spence

Operations & Finance
Operations Director Jacqui Kell
Finance Manager Antony Robertson
Finance Officer Catherine Moody

Development
Director Development & Enterprise Lucy Bird
Development Manager Caitrin Innis

Marketing & Communications
Marketing & Communications Manager Cait Read
Marketing & Communications Officer (Digital) Lisa Campbell
Marketing & Communications Officer (CRM & Data) Kate Stacey

Charlotte Josephine

POPS

OBERON BOOKS
LONDON

WWW.OBERONBOOKS.COM

First published in 2019 by Oberon Books Ltd
521 Caledonian Road, London N7 9RH
Tel: +44 (0) 20 7607 3637 / Fax: +44 (0) 20 7607 3629
e-mail: info@oberonbooks.com
www.oberonbooks.com

PB ISBN: 9781786828422
E ISBN: 9781786828439

Cover photo by Bronwen Sharp
Artwork by Rebecca Pitt

Printed and bound by 4EDGE Limited, Hockley, Essex, UK.
eBook conversion by Lapiz Digital Services, India.

10 9 8 7 6 5 4 3 2 1

Cast

NOTE: Stage directions are in italics and brackets. Capital letters are used to suggest an emphasis on specific words.

A / indicates a fast run onto the next line, almost an interruption.

A /.. indicates where a word can't be found and something physical happens instead. Perhaps it's a small naturalistic gesture or perhaps a big abstract movement, each one is an invitation to express something physically.

A * indicates a new scene. A shift in tone.

*DAUGHTER: I won't stay for long. I promise.

FATHER: It's fine!

DAUGHTER: Be out of your hair/

FATHER: there's no/

DAUGHTER: as soon as/

FATHER: honestly, there's no/

DAUGHTER: I just need to/..

FATHER: Get back on your feet.

DAUGHTER: Exactly.

FATHER: .

DAUGHTER: I/

FATHER: honestly, it's no/..

DAUGHTER: I'm really grateful.

FATHER: Well it's. Really, the least I/..

> *(Silence. It's awkward. Neither of them knows what to do. A lot is not said. He looks about the room, points to the telly, 'Come Dine With Me' is on. He sits down to watch it.)*

FATHER: I love this.

DAUGHTER: .

FATHER: Come and sit down!

> *(She does, though she doesn't want to. It's hot in this room. He doesn't take his eyes off the television as he talks to her.)*

DAUGHTER: How's your day been?

FATHER: Oh tickety boo tickety boo. Not bad for a
    Wednesday.

DAUGHTER: It's Thursday.

FATHER: Is it?

DAUGHTER: Yeah.

FATHER: Oh! I've lost one!

(He laughs, she doesn't.)

FATHER: I love this.

DAUGHTER: .

FATHER: Ooooh she's a bitch that one!

DAUGHTER: .

FATHER: I'd do roast beef.

DAUGHTER: .

FATHER: Can't go wrong with a Good Roast Beef.

DAUGHTER: Unless you're vegetarian.

FATHER: Which no one *really* is.

DAUGHTER: No?

FATHER: Not *really*.

DAUGHTER: .

FATHER: Yeah. Roast beef. Or that Pork Dish.

DAUGHTER: .

FATHER: .

DAUGHTER: What pork dish?

FATHER: That Pork Dish I used to/

DAUGHTER: don't remember a/

FATHER: don't you *remember*?

DAUGHTER: No/

FATHER: I used to do a Pork Dish, don't you/

DAUGHTER: no/

FATHER: *remember*? This *lovely* Pork Dish/

DAUGHTER: no/

FATHER: you used to *love* that/

DAUGHTER: I don't/

FATHER: you used to *guzzle* it down/

DAUGHTER: I don't /

FATHER: no? Oh, you used to *love* that!

DAUGHTER: .

FATHER: What about you?

DAUGHTER: What about me?

FATHER: What would you do? Not a Pork Dish.

DAUGHTER: No, not a Pork Dish.

FATHER: No.

DAUGHTER: No. Because I'm a vegetarian.

FATHER: No!

DAUGHTER: Yes. I did say I/

FATHER: yeah but you're not *really* a/

DAUGHTER: yes, I am.

FATHER: No one's *really* a/

DAUGHTER: yes, they are.

FATHER: Just *silly*! No one's *really*/

DAUGHTER: yes they are! *I am!*

FATHER: .

DAUGHTER: .

FATHER: He's a wally that one.

DAUGHTER: .

FATHER: Reminds me of old what's his name.

DAUGHTER: .

FATHER: What's his name?

DAUGHTER: Who/

FATHER: you know/

DAUGHTER: no/

FATHER: you know! From the school! Bloody. What's his name?!

DAUGHTER: Who?

FATHER: Your teacher! The posh one. Oh! What's his/

DAUGHTER: Mr Heggerty/

FATHER: Heggerty! Heggerty! Hegger-ty. With his/.. And his /.. Always so/..

8

(They proper crack up laughing. We have no idea why, but it's joyful to watch. They eventually stop, they sigh in the same way. She smiles, watching him watching the telly. Without taking his eyes off the telly he reaches across to the cassette player and presses play. An old song plays softly. She stares at it, suddenly feels sick.)

FATHER: Oh, blimey I/

DAUGHTER: it's fine!

FATHER: I didn't think I/

DAUGHTER: honestly, it's cool/

FATHER: you don't mind?

DAUGHTER: No no no it's fine/

FATHER: sorry/

DAUGHTER: no/

FATHER: stupid/

DAUGHTER: it's fine!

FATHER: I love this….It's proper….Rock n roll.

(She nods trying not to look at the cassette player. Without taking his eyes off the telly he turns the volume up on the cassette player one notch. Her body shudders.)

FATHER: So, not a Roast Beef.

DAUGHTER: No.

FATHER: No! Roast, nut, thing? Nut roast?

9

DAUGHTER: Yeah, maybe. Yeah, or, maybe a, erm.

FATHER: Yeah?

DAUGHTER: .

FATHER: Yeah?

DAUGHTER: Dunno.

FATHER: No, go on.

DAUGHTER: Can't think/

FATHER: go on!

DAUGHTER: Really. I dunno/

FATHER: don't get all/

DAUGHTER: I'm not! I'm just, it's fine, it's.

(They sit in silence. He turns the volume up again. She shuts her eyes as he does it, grips the chair tighter. They watch the telly. He reaches for the cassette player again.)

DAUGHTER: How can you/

FATHER: what/

DAUGHTER: both. At the same time.

FATHER: It's fine.

DAUGHTER: But you can't hear/

FATHER: it's Fine. It's how I like it.

(He wants to turn it up again. He doesn't, but she feels it anyway. She watches him. He watches the TV.)

FATHER: It's Great you're back.

DAUGHTER: Yeah.

FATHER: Yeah!

(He reaches for the volume but stops short, turns the reach into a dance move. He bops along to the music shyly, trying to lighten the mood. She can't look at him, is embarrassed by something. She stays for as long as she can bear it.)

DAUGHTER: I'm gonna/..

FATHER: Oh, ok.

DAUGHTER: I'm really tired.

FATHER: Of course, of course. Yeah course, you must be. I'll keep it down low/

DAUGHTER: you don't have to/

FATHER: don't want to disturb/

DAUGHTER: no please, just, do what you'd normally do. I don't want to/

FATHER: you're not!

DAUGHTER: Ok, cool.

FATHER: Cool.

DAUGHTER: Night then.

(He goes to move towards her but she has already left, taking her big bags with her.)

FATHER: Night sweetheart.

(He sits in his chair, alone. He gently bobs along to the music. The song finishes; he sits still for a moment, staring into space. He looks at the door she has just left through. He looks at the cassette player. He replays the song.)

*(The television is on, the blue light flickering around the room, cold and lonely. She enters and stands for a moment watching him. He is sat in his chair watching 'Come Dine With Me' on television. The cassette player is on, the song playing softly in the background. She puts a smile on her lips and a cheery tone in her voice. She steps forward and he suddenly notices her.)

FATHER: *(Big smile.)* Hiya love!

DAUGHTER: *(Small smile.)* Hiya.

FATHER: Come and sit down!

(The blue light flickers on their faces.)

FATHER: *(Big smile.)* Hiya love!

DAUGHTER: *(Small smile.)* Hiya.

FATHER: Come and sit down!

(The blue light flickers on their faces.)

FATHER: *(Big smile.)* Hiya love!

DAUGHTER: *(Small smile.)* Hiya.

FATHER: Come and sit down!

(The blue light flickers on their faces.)

FATHER: *(Big smile.)* Hiya love!

DAUGHTER: What's that?

FATHER: Hot chocolate.

DAUGHTER: .

FATHER: I made it for you/

DAUGHTER: why?

FATHER: You like it.

DAUGHTER: .

FATHER: You used to like/

DAUGHTER: I'm twenty-nine years old.

(The blue light flickers on their faces.)

FATHER: Hiya love!

DAUGHTER: Hiya.

FATHER: Come and sit down!

(The blue light flickers on their faces.)

FATHER: Hiya love!

DAUGHTER: Hiya.

FATHER: Come and sit down!

(The blue light flickers on their faces.)

FATHER: Hiya love!

DAUGHTER: Hiya.

FATHER: Come and sit down!

(The blue light flickers on their faces.)

FATHER: Hiya love.

DAUGHTER: *Fuck!*

FATHER: What's wrong/

DAUGHTER: just. Fuck!

FATHER: Sweetheart/

DAUGHTER: *Fuuuuuuck!* I've had a fucking Shit fucking day alright?! Literally fucking Nothing's gone right and everyone, fucking Everyone's a fucking cunt and I just need to fucking Chill, the Fuck, Out, and I don't even. Fuck! How d'you? *Fuck!* And as soon as I get in the Fucking Door you're all, *There*, in my *face?!*

FATHER: .

DAUGHTER: .

FATHER: .

DAUGHTER: Sorry.

(The blue light flickers on their faces.)

FATHER: *(Big smile.)* Hiya love!

DAUGHTER: Hiya.

FATHER: Come and sit down!

14

(The blue light flickers on their faces.)

FATHER: Hiya love!

DAUGHTER: Hiya.

FATHER: Come and sit down!

(The blue light flickers on their faces.)

FATHER: Hiya love!

DAUGHTER: Hiya.

FATHER: Come and/

> *(He is suddenly visibly upset. His hand is bleeding. She's never seen him like this.)*

DAUGHTER: Dad! What have you done?

FATHER: I cut it/

DAUGHTER: what?

FATHER: Washing up and it just, smashed, in my hand I/

DAUGHTER: Fuck! Here I'll/

FATHER: just trying to do the, can't even do/

DAUGHTER: it's ok, it's/

FATHER: useless aren't I?

DAUGHTER: No Dad of course you're/

FATHER: useless. Completely. *Useless!*

DAUGHTER: Stop it/

FATHER: fucking *Pathetic!*

15

DAUGHTER: Stop it Dad you're scaring me!

FATHER: Oh sorry! Sorry, sorry. Sorry,
    sorrrrrysorrysorrysorry/

DAUGHTER: Dad/

FATHER: sorrysorrrrysorryyyysorrysorry/

DAUGHTER: Dad! Stop it!

FATHER: Shhhhhhhh!

DAUGHTER: .

(The blue light flickers on their faces.)

FATHER: *(Big smile.)* Hiya love!

DAUGHTER: *(Little smile.)* Hiya.

FATHER: Come and sit down!

(The blue light flickers on their faces. He feels the audience watching him.)

FATHER: *(To her and us.)* Hiya love.

DAUGHTER: Hiya.

FATHER: *(To her.)* Come and/.. *(To us.)* I'm going to say it. Just
    come straight out and. And she won't want to hear it but
    that's tough because it Needs to be said it's Time. And
    she'll probably cry, because that's what she does, and I'll
    probably get angry and/.. But because I've actually Said
    it then/.. She'll Apologise, she'll have to. And then I will,
    and for once we'll mean it and, it won't be Sorted straight
    away of course it. But it'll be a Start, it'll be/

DAUGHTER: alright?

FATHER: *(To her.)* Alright.

DAUGHTER: .

FATHER: Come and sit down. She's cooked this carbonara thing. Looks bloody awful. And the commentator, that's not the right word, the, whatever you know what I, well he's proper laying into her.

DAUGHTER: Dad?

FATHER: Proper laying into her all like. Emcee, is that it?

DAUGHTER: Dad?

FATHER: The Emcee. He's proper laying into her.

DAUGHTER: Dad?

FATHER: Going *oooh yes Julie, that looks delightful* when it bloody doesn't.

DAUGHTER: Dad?

FATHER: And she's all Proud of herself, dishing this Slop up on the table like it's Gordon bloody Ramsay or something.

DAUGHTER: Dad?

FATHER: Like it's gourmet.

DAUGHTER: Dad.

FATHER: This Slop? And they're all looking at it, looking at this Slop like *Jesus! Sweet Jesus, don't make me eat that shit!*

DAUGHTER: Dad.

FATHER: But they're all too polite, that's people's these days. Everyone's Too Polite.

DAUGHTER: Dad.

FATHER: No one really says what they mean.

DAUGHTER: Dad.

FATHER: So they eat it. They'd actually rather Eat It, than be Honest? Astounding really. That's social conditioning that.

DAUGHTER: Dad.

FATHER: Astounding.

DAUGHTER: Dad.

FATHER: What love?

DAUGHTER: /..

FATHER: Hiya love!

DAUGHTER: Hiya.

FATHER: Come and/

DAUGHTER: the bus was late and I'm trying not to panic because that doesn't really help does it? I mean, it doesn't exactly make it come any faster.

FATHER: Love?

DAUGHTER: Me standing there, being annoyed at it doesn't make it come any faster. And I thought/

FATHER: love?

DAUGHTER: Should I walk? Should I just walk it? I mean I'm gonna be late anyway/

FATHER: love?

DAUGHTER: And it's quite a nice day so maybe I should just walk.

FATHER: Love?

DAUGHTER: But I didn't wanna turn up all sweaty. You know when your T-shirt sticks to you?

FATHER: Love?

DAUGHTER: Gross. Not a good first impression eh? And then, *eventually,* it turns up, like *twenty-seven* minutes late.

FATHER: Love?

DAUGHTER: *Twenty-Seven Minutes Late?*

FATHER: Love?

DAUGHTER: And I get on and it's only then that I realize, I've left my bloody purse at home. By the front door so I wouldn't forget it. And *still* somehow I've bloody/

FATHER: *(To us.)* love.

DAUGHTER: Stupid.

FATHER: *(To us.)* Love.

DAUGHTER: So *stupid!*

FATHER: *(To us.)* Love.

DAUGHTER: And then the bloody bloke wouldn't let me get on! I said, *Oi yeah I get this bus everyday mate every fucking day* and yeah alright maybe I shouldn't have sworn but/

FATHER: *(To her.)* love.

DAUGHTER: it just fucking, *fuck! Sorry, listen I'll pay you back tomorrow* but he's having none of it. Said he'll call the police if I don't get off and *Alright mate! Take it easy, I'm getting off, fucksake! Meant to be a Public service?! Can't even make a simple mistake?!*

FATHER: Love.

DAUGHTER: Fucksake.

FATHER: Love.

DAUGHTER: Yeah?

FATHER: /..

DAUGHTER: .

FATHER: .

DAUGHTER: .

FATHER: We could get chips from the shop up the/

DAUGHTER: I think I'm gonna apply for it/

FATHER: they're the best round here now/

DAUGHTER: they've had the notice up for over a week/

FATHER: used to be Rosie's up by the pub/

DAUGHTER: just a few days a week/

FATHER: lovely that was/

DAUGHTER: just part time/

FATHER: roll out at closing time/

DAUGHTER: don't think I could/

FATHER: and get a bag from Rosie's/

DAUGHTER: more than part time/

FATHER: no good now. Changed their oil I think/

DAUGHTER: think it'd be good for me/

FATHER: no they're no good now/

DAUGHTER: you're not/

FATHER: what/

DAUGHTER: listening/

FATHER: you're not/

DAUGHTER: what/

FATHER: listening.

(They look at each other for a beat, then back to the telly.)

DAUGHTER: Build my confidence/

FATHER: shame really/

DAUGHTER: bit by bit/

FATHER: used to be lovely/

DAUGHTER: baby steps/

FATHER: best in town now/

DAUGHTER: baby steps/

FATHER: is that new one up the road.

(He turns up the volume on the cassette player one notch. She shudders. The blue light flickers on their faces. He turns up the volume another notch. She snaps.)

DAUGHTER: Is it everyday?

FATHER: What?

DAUGHTER: It's everyday.

FATHER: *(To us.)* No it's/

DAUGHTER: yes it is!

FATHER: *(To us.)* So? *(To her.)* So what? I like it. What's wrong with/

DAUGHTER: you know what's/

FATHER: I'm fine, it's fine.

FATHER: It's Fine.

(He doesn't want to but he has to turn up the volume on the cassette player. Is compelled to. Without taking his eyes off the telly he turns it up one notch. He looks at her. She is looking straight back at him. There's a moment where they see themselves in each other, and it's the most terrifying thing they have ever seen. He looks away. She slowly gets up from her chair to look closer at him. He doesn't seem to notice, transfixed by the telly. She reaches out to touch her dad's cheek. As soon as she makes contact she snap sits back down and watches the television. He looks at the cassette player, looks at it like he's not looked at it in years, like something about it is suddenly new to him. She doesn't take her eyes off the television but she feels the compulsion in him. He leans over to the cassette player and turns up the volume one notch. He turns it up quite a few notches. It's loud. It's too loud. They both ignore it and watch the television. The blue light flickers on their faces. He smiles as he speaks to us. She doesn't seem to notice.)

FATHER: Back in them days there was a community, a real sense of. Not like now, not like/.. All the lads together, clock in, all jokes and back slaps and. Golden. Golden days. Not like now, now it's/.. I didn't quit! I'm not a quitter! I know that's what you, people think don't they, just scum. Don't bother with the likes of, don't Help them, oh no, dirty scum. Greedy, lazy, fucking, Stupid no good Fucking layabouts, cheating the system? Think I'm stupid think I'm/

(She suddenly exits. He watches her go. He speaks to us.)

FATHER: She gives me this Look sometimes. I see her. Looking at me. Like she's, looking at me like I'm/

(The blue light flickers on his face.)

22

(She enters with a tray. He looks back at the telly. A glass of water and a plate of salad are on the tray. She eats slowly and mindfully. He watches her, snorts once and shakes his head. She doesn't look across to him but pauses in her eating to speak to him.)

DAUGHTER: What?

FATHER: Nothing.

(She eats. He watches television.)

FATHER: Horses eat that.

(She shrugs, but the comment hurt. He looks confused as to why he said it. They sit in silence in front of the TV. Her phone beeps. He turns to her, curious. She replies to the text, smiling. He turns back to the TV. Her phone beeps again. He looks at her. She is smiling reading the phone. He looks back to the TV. Her phone beeps. He tries not to look at her. It beeps again. He tries not to look. It beeps again and he can't help himself.)

FATHER: A boy?

DAUGHTER: What?

FATHER: Is that a/

DAUGHTER: no/

FATHER: got you smiling like that/

DAUGHTER: no/

FATHER: blushing like that/

DAUGHTER: no/

FATHER: make sure he pays for dinner.

23

DAUGHTER: What?!

FATHER: He should pay.

(She opens her mouth but has nothing to say. They both look away to the TV. They sit in silence. He turns up the volume on the cassette player one notch and she shudders. He looks at her, maybe he saw the shudder. They stare at the TV. She stands.)

FATHER: Where are you/

DAUGHTER: you know where I'm/

FATHER: meetings meetings meetings. Meetings meetings. Meetings meetings meetings meetings. Meet/

DAUGHTER: would you like to come.

(He snorts. She turns to leave.)

FATHER: Waste of bloody time. Sitting around Moaning about their lives.

DAUGHTER: That's not really/

FATHER: talking about God? There ain't a God!

DAUGHTER: Ok/

FATHER: and that's a Fact, that's a fucking Fact!

DAUGHTER: Ok.

FATHER: You tell 'em that from me.

DAUGHTER: Alright.

FATHER: Tell 'em that's a Fucking Fact!

(She leaves. He turns the volume up really loud. He sits muttering to himself. Dances a little. Suddenly turns to us.)

FATHER: Oh yeah. Oh yeah, she's probably waiting, for me to, but She's the one! It's got to, She was the one who/.. She's/..She's stubborn. Just like her mother so bloody, just can't admit it when she's, if she would just Own up to it then we could, Move and, Fresh start but. I'll talk to her. I will, I'll tell her/

DAUGHTER: alright?

FATHER: .

DAUGHTER: What you doing today?

FATHER: Nothing.

DAUGHTER: Oh. That's a shame/

FATHER: is it?

DAUGHTER: It's a beautiful day!

FATHER: Is it?

DAUGHTER: Yes! Yeah, it's/..

FATHER: What?

DAUGHTER: Glorious.

FATHER: "Glorious".

DAUGHTER: Yes. It's a *glorious* day... The birds are singing, the sun is shining, the sky is blue, blue blue. Oh! I would drink that sky if I could/

FATHER: of course you would/

DAUGHTER: what?

FATHER: If you could/

DAUGHTER: so/

FATHER: but you can't so/

DAUGHTER: so?

(She frowns at him. He smiles at her. He's won.)

DAUGHTER: One day I'll have a house of my own.

FATHER: Not likely. Not at these prices.

DAUGHTER: I want to lay in my bed with a book, and a cup of tea, and out of the window is green green green. And lay in my bath, and out the steamy window is sky sky sky. And stand at my kitchen sink, doing the washing up, humming some old song because I feel, Quietly Content. And out of the window will be a tree. And I will watch that tree grow, and change, watch the leaves turn from green to orange, fall and stand bare. But I'll feel safe knowing they're gonna grow back, green and new, and I don't have to do a thing. That tree? Will grow without me grow *beautifully*, without me I don't have to shout at the leaves, *grow, grow!* They will, in their own time, the way they were meant to whether I'm here or not. I'll look out my window and/

FATHER: you'll be lucky. House prices round here are through the roof.

(She watches him watching the television. The cassette player is playing softly in the background.)

26

FATHER: Come and sit down!

DAUGHTER: Can't.

FATHER: Oh?

DAUGHTER: Got that interview.

FATHER: .

DAUGHTER: Dad. Dad. I've got an interview! For that job I/

FATHER: think I've seen this one.

DAUGHTER: .

FATHER: What love?

DAUGHTER: Nothing.

(She leaves. He turns up the cassette player one notch. Exhales. Turns it up another notch. Exhales. He reaches to turn it up again but it does it itself. He finds this amusing, starts a little dance in his chair. Points at the cassette player and it gets louder. He dances bigger in his chair. Points at the cassette player and it gets louder. Speaks to us over the music.)

FATHER: When I met her she had this yellow dress on.
Yellow? Yellow?! I mean, who wears yellow for Christ
sake?! But she looked gorgeous of course she, she was
Gorgeous, I told her, walked Straight over and said *You,
are gorgeous.* Couldn't believe I, I mean, me? Who did I
think I?! But she smiled, this smile, this. We danced, all
night we/.. Music was great then, was Great! Was Proper
you know? Not like now not like/..

(The music gets louder and he is compelled to stand up and dance. It's wonderful to watch him moving, cheeky and fun. He shows us his moves.)

FATHER: We'd do this/.. And this one/.. Give 'em one of these/..

(It gets more wild and the music starts to stutter and skip. She enters and watches him dancing. He's in his own world and starting to get out of control. She becomes aware of us, is embarrassed we're seeing them like this. She calls out to him to slow down, to stop. He ignores her. She suddenly turns and speaks to us. He continues to dance all over the stage, oblivious to her. She stands impossibly still, holding on.)

DAUGHTER: I tried to get there early. Because they say on time is late right? So I tried to be like, ten minutes early, give myself time to, get settled you know, calm. But I couldn't decide what to wear and left the house late and forgot my purse again and missed the bus and had to run into town. Up that big hill. And got there all sweaty and panting and my heart doing that thing that, tight chest thing I, *sorry sorry I'm, sorry I'm here for the, for the, I'm not Late am I?* And the woman on the desk looked at me like, this Look like, like I'm some dirty pathetic scummy piece of shitbag and why am I even bothering I might as well just go and Die, go and die somewhere, quietly, out of peoples way. She points, this manicure fucking perfect posh fucking finger point and, I go in and. I dunno. I try my best but... *Well I really Care about erm, hospitality and, I would enjoy the opportunity to erm, be of service and you know, serve, the servers, the customers the.* Shit... *Yes, for, a while now yes. Erm, health reasons. All sorted now yes.* No. Fuck. *No, sorry I don't have a reference. They erm. They're not very, nice, people, I was a Good worker there I was really, trying I. I. No, thank you.* Fuck!

(She shame-scream-squirms. She stops. She looks at her dad who's still dancing. She calmly walks over and gently stops him. He's exhausted, keeps muttering 'sorry love'. She helps him sit in his chair. She checks his airway is clear. Once he's settled she stands still, tired.)

(The lights snap up and he sits upright. A new day.)

FATHER: Hiya love!

DAUGHTER: *(Weakly.)* Hiya.

FATHER: Come and sit down!

DAUGHTER: .

FATHER: How'd it go?

   (She shrugs.)

FATHER: What does/

DAUGHTER: I didn't get it.

FATHER: Oh.

DAUGHTER: Yeah.

FATHER: Well.

DAUGHTER: .

FATHER: Well. Fuck 'em! Eh? Fuck 'em!

DAUGHTER: .

FATHER: And, what about? The doctors. Did you/

DAUGHTER: I'm on a waiting list/

FATHER: great. Ok. Great! That's, great.

DAUGHTER: .

FATHER: How long will/

DAUGHTER: at least six months/

FATHER: six *months?*

DAUGHTER: At least.

FATHER: .

DAUGHTER: Yeah.

FATHER: Ok. Ok. Ok/

DAUGHTER: ok?

FATHER: Well. You probably don't, need, it anyway. You were just, checking weren't you? If you Needed, which you probably don't so. Just. You'll be fine, we'll be fine.

DAUGHTER: .

(He turns the volume up a notch. She shudders. She stares at him. He feels her looking.)

FATHER: What?

DAUGHTER: Do you have to/

FATHER: what? I'm enjoying myself.

(She laughs at him.)

FATHER: Can't a man enjoy himself? In his own home/

DAUGHTER: your level of denial/

FATHER: oh! And you're sorted aren't you/

DAUGHTER: it's astounding/

FATHER: you're so Sorted/

DAUGHTER: really it's/

FATHER: you're *cured!*

DAUGHTER: I never said I/

FATHER: don't you *ever* dictate to me/

DAUGHTER: I'm not dictat/

FATHER: just cus you've joined a Cult!

DAUGHTER: Wow! Ok?! Wow!

FATHER: Walking around like some bloody born again
   Christian/

DAUGHTER: right/

FATHER: judging me?

DAUGHTER: ok/

FATHER: telling *me* what to do?

DAUGHTER: I've never told/

FATHER: judging people who just want to have a Good time,
   who want to have fun/

DAUGHTER: oh! Is that what you think you're doing?!
   Really?!

   (He giggles.)

FATHER: When did you get so/

DAUGHTER: what/

FATHER: so Serious all the/

DAUGHTER: it is Serious! It's Really Serious!

(He laughs. She gets annoyed.)

FATHER: Oh come on! Lighten up!

DAUGHTER: You're a joke. This whole, you're a fucking joke/

FATHER: don't swear! I am your Father/

DAUGHTER: yeah?

FATHER: Yeah. I may not be perfect/

DAUGHTER: no/

FATHER: but I *am* trying.

DAUGHTER: Are you?

FATHER: Yes.

DAUGHTER: Shame, cus it still ain't good enough.

FATHER: Oh well! Ok. Ok. Ok! Yeah you win. Fine. I'll just, that's fine/

DAUGHTER: Dad/

FATHER: don't worry about it/

DAUGHTER: Dad I/

FATHER: no no, don't worry about it.

DAUGHTER: I'm, I'm gonna/

FATHER: ok.

(She waits. He won't look at her. He turns the volume up a few notches. He dances, eyes closed, in his own world. She's about to

leave but instead runs to stand on a chair. She speaks to us over the
music, the speech pours out of her before she can stop it.)

DAUGHTER: It's Sunday morning and the church bells are
   ringing, ringing ringing but I'm not going. I'm stuck, to
   cold tiles tip toeing like a child though I am no longer
   child I am woman, I suppose, though often I'm not sure
   what that means.

   Stuck, to cold tiles barefoot and bleary eyed. Sleepy
   morning toes fidget and flex, wondering where's the tea 'n'
   toast they were promised if they got out of bed? Made it
   downstairs but daren't take another step, stuck at the edge
   of the room.

   There's a whale beached on the kitchen floor.

   White tiles, bleached and cold reflect steamed breath
   each time it snores and oh, how it snores. A clogged roar,
   terrifying, and solemn. Mucus like seaweed caught on its
   tongue threatens to choke its throat on each swell of the
   tide. I wonder how it's still alive? Each wave shakes my
   insides, my rib cage vibrates, the back of my teeth actually
   ache its roar rattles right fucking through me.

   It's been here before, washed up on the shore unwanted
   and unwelcome. I tip toe through puddles, praying it
   doesn't wake doesn't startle and shake wondering how on
   earth, under what stars, what crimes moonlight watched
   it perform last night. Forcing the sea to spit him out onto
   shore, onto cold fucking floor that on a weekday is *spotless!*
   But at the weekend? Beached. Half drowned himself.

FATHER: Love?

DAUGHTER: Salty seawater clogs up your blow 'oles/

FATHER: love.

DAUGHTER: Kettle clicks. Black, two sugars/

FATHER: love.

DAUGHTER: Sip slow, Dad. It's Sunday morning. The church, it's the church bells ringing, ringing ringing. But neither of us is going.

(He stops dancing. She is tired. He looks out at us.)

FATHER: Hiya love!

DAUGHTER: . *(She is still looking at us.)*

FATHER: Come and sit down!

(Without taking his eyes off the telly he reaches across to the cassette player and turns up the volume a notch. She watches him do it. She stands right in front of the television. He doesn't seem to notice, watching it through her like she's sat next to him. She walks behind the television and pulls the back off it easily. She climbs inside the television and watches her dad through it. He doesn't seem to notice. Her phone beeps from the armchair. She closes her eyes. It beeps again. She puts her hands over her ears. It beeps twice more. He points at it without taking his eyes off the television.)

FATHER: It's that boy again.

(She opens her eyes and speaks to us.)

DAUGHTER: I am standing waiting for him. And it is raining it is raining it is raining. And he is late, but it's ok I've already forgiven him he'll be here soon, he will. He'll be here soon, running towards me apologizing for being so late. And I'm smiling telling him it's ok it's ok, it's ok. And he holds me and I smile. And he kisses me kisses me

34

kisses me. And I feel like this time, This Time. I won't
Want, Too Much. And he won't Want, Too Little. We will
Want each other in Equal Amounts and it will be good. It
will be Good, it Will be Good.

FATHER: He didn't turn up.

*(She smiles to stop herself from crying. She shakes her head, smiling.
She shrugs, smiling. Smiling.)*

FATHER: Fuck him! Plenty more fish in the sea.

DAUGHTER: Yeah?

FATHER: Yeah!

DAUGHTER: I'm sick of the sea. I'm drowning.

*(He looks at her. He turns off the cassette player. The silence is
startling. She climbs out of the television. They look at each other.)*

FATHER: Men are shit.

DAUGHTER: Yeah. Yeah they are.

(They laugh.)

FATHER: Going to one of your meet/

DAUGHTER: no, I/

FATHER: oh, ok.

DAUGHTER: Think I'm gonna, run a bath?

FATHER: Ok.

DAUGHTER: That ok?

FATHER: Yeah! 'course. There's that, stuff that/

DAUGHTER: Radox. Thanks.

FATHER: Ok.

(She goes to leave. She turns back and kisses her dad softly on his forehead.)

FATHER: Ok.

(He stares into space, smiling. She leaves. He sits quietly, smiling. He looks at the cassette player.)

(Silence. The cassette player is gone. She enters and notices instantly. She smiles at her dad. They sit together. Smiling in silence.)

(They make a cup of tea together. They barely speak as they boil a kettle, brew, pour, and drink the tea. It takes as long as it takes. It's lovely to witness, quiet and simple.)

DAUGHTER: Because people just aren't kind anymore.

FATHER: That's right!

DAUGHTER: Not like they used to be, not/

TOGETHER: Consistently.

(They smile.)

FATHER: That's right. That's right.

DAUGHTER: Like some One-Off good deed is enough? But it's Not it's, it's really just the little things/

FATHER: the little things/

DAUGHTER: lots of Little things/

FATHER: that make all the difference. It's the ants that get ya/

DAUGHTER: not the elephants! They said that at/.. In the/.. They said/

FATHER: it's the ants/

DAUGHTER: yeah/

FATHER: not the elephants. Not the big things. The Little everyday/

DAUGHTER: yes/

FATHER: smile at a stranger. Hold a door open/

DAUGHTER: talk to the person behind the counter/

FATHER: no one talks anymore/

DAUGHTER: no one really listens/

FATHER: all got bloody headphones in/

DAUGHTER: yeah/

FATHER: well, it's Fear isn't it.

DAUGHTER: Yeah!

FATHER: Don't look at each other/

DAUGHTER: head down get on with it/

FATHER: selfish. Just thinking about me and mine? Fucking Tories!

DAUGHTER: Yes!

FATHER: Closing down community centres/

DAUGHTER: cutting the NHS/

FATHER: old people? Young people? All fucked/

DAUGHTER: mental health takes the hardest/

FATHER: nowhere for people to go/

DAUGHTER: on a waiting list forever. They don't care.

FATHER: Course not. Fuck the Tories!

DAUGHTER: Fuck the Tories!

FATHER: Just cruel. No one's kind anymore, and it ripples out you know? You've got to Try, try to be kind, consistent kindness.

(She smiles at him then drinks her tea. He watches her, smiling.)

FATHER: Been thinking.

DAUGHTER: Oh?

FATHER: 'bout clearing that old shed out. Make some space to, do your painting or whatever it is you, do you still do that?

DAUGHTER: No. Not really/

FATHER: oh, well/

DAUGHTER: no! I mean, I'd like to! Yes, please, that'd be nice.

FATHER: Ok.

DAUGHTER: Ok.

FATHER: 'bout time I did some work in the garden too. I've neglected it.

DAUGHTER: Get your green fingers on?

FATHER: That's right. That's right.

(They smile at each other. Then she is suddenly shy.)

DAUGHTER: D'you remember, at Christmas, years ago, when we made a snowman?

FATHER: Yeah. You bossing me about/

DAUGHTER: I wasn't!

FATHER: You were!

DAUGHTER: *"You do the body, I'll do the head."*

FATHER: Your fingers went blue. Didn't have gloves on/

DAUGHTER: didn't matter. Still had a good/

FATHER: I forgot them/

DAUGHTER: Mum went mad/

FATHER: no.

DAUGHTER: .

FATHER: She'd left by then.

DAUGHTER: No.

FATHER: .

DAUGHTER: She left in/

FATHER: October.

DAUGHTER: No.

FATHER: October/

DAUGHTER: can't have. She was there! I remember/

FATHER: no.

DAUGHTER: I remember/

FATHER: no.

DAUGHTER: I remember *specifically/*

FATHER: No! You've remembered it wrong.

DAUGHTER: .

FATHER: It's ok. It happens, it's/..

> *(Silence. They suddenly can't look at each other. Whatever it is that's not said is painful. She looks up and catches him looking at the door.)*

FATHER: You ok?

DAUGHTER: Yeah?

FATHER: You seem a bit/

DAUGHTER: no/

FATHER: bit, Tense.

DAUGHTER: No, I'm fine/

FATHER: ok.

DAUGHTER: Ok.

> *(They both look at the door, then back to each other.)*

DAUGHTER: Look at you!

FATHER: What?

DAUGHTER: You're practically/

FATHER: no I'm/

DAUGHTER: practically Crawling/

FATHER: I'm fine.

DAUGHTER: *(To us.)* Crawling with it.

FATHER: *(To us.)* I'm fine! You're the one who/

DAUGHTER: *(To us.)* I'm fine.

FATHER: *(Laughs.)* Oh! Yeah/

DAUGHTER: *(To him.)* I am actually. *(To us.)* I'm actually really fine/

FATHER: *(To us.)* Oh yeah!

DAUGHTER: I'm great. I am I'm, *(To him.)* I'm doing great/

FATHER: *(To us.)* great!

DAUGHTER: *(To us.)* I'm going to a meeting.

FATHER: *(To us.)* Great.

DAUGHTER: *(To him.)* Perhaps you'd like to come?

(He laughs at her. She stares at him.)

DAUGHTER: What?

FATHER: You think, you Actually think/

DAUGHTER: no/

FATHER: you do, you Actually think you're Better than me/

DAUGHTER: no/

FATHER: fucking, Better, than Me?

DAUGHTER: Ok, you're getting hostile.

FATHER: Blood runs thicker. *(To us.)* Can't escape it. Dress it up in whatever pretty language you want but scratch the surface and we're the same/

DAUGHTER: *(To us.)* ok this is/

FATHER: *(To us.)* we're the *same!*

DAUGHTER: *(To him.)* Why can't you just/

FATHER: *(To her.)* what/

DAUGHTER: apologise!

FATHER: Hah! You first.

DAUGHTER: *(To everyone.)* Ok. This isn't working/

FATHER: *(To everyone.)* clearly.

DAUGHTER: I'm going to/

FATHER: good, good. Meeting/

DAUGHTER: meeting.

FATHER: Meeting. Good, that's good.

DAUGHTER: .

FATHER: *(To her.)* They work?

DAUGHTER: *(To everyone.)* Hope so.

> *(She exits. He paces, mutters to himself, tries to calm himself, turns and turns and turns. He speaks to us.)*

FATHER: She used to fit along my arm, here. Her whole body, the length of my arm. Wrist to elbow. Head to toe. A whole body, a life, so wonderful, so/..

(The music suddenly blares loud. He holds his ears and sways, terrified. The music suddenly muffles in volume. He speaks to us.)

FATHER: I wake up on the floor, again. And I have no idea I/.. I don't?/.. The floor is hard and cold and I can feel all of my, skeleton? Trying to be hard and cold, trying to/.. But something is rubbing my back? Softly, softly and I know it is her. And I fucking want her to fucking stop, I'm trying my best to/..

(The music suddenly blares loud and he dances. Violently thrashing. She enters and watches him. He is startled but can't stop thrashing. The music dips in volume and they speak to us, competing for our approval. His body continues to thrash involuntarily sometimes. She is stood impossibly still.)

DAUGHTER: It's Sunday morning and the church bells are ringing/

FATHER: I wake up on the floor, again/

DAUGHTER: ringing ringing but we're not going, we're not fucking/

FATHER: and I have no idea I. I don't/

DAUGHTER: stuck, to cold tiles/

FATHER: fuck/

DAUGHTER: though I am no longer/

FATHER: the floor is hard/

DAUGHTER: I am woman, I suppose/

FATHER: hard and cold/

DAUGHTER: not sure what that means/

FATHER: I can feel all of my, skeleton?

DAUGHTER: Trying to be/

FATHER: trying to/

DAUGHTER: stuck, barefoot and bleary eyed.

FATHER: Something is rubbing my back?

DAUGHTER: Softly softly, stuck/

FATHER: and I know it is Her.

DAUGHTER: There's a Whale beached on the kitchen floor/

FATHER: and I fucking want her to fucking stop/

DAUGHTER: each time it snores and oh, how it snores/

FATHER: stop/

DAUGHTER: a clogged roar/

FATHER: stop/

DAUGHTER: terrifying, and solemn/

FATHER: fucking stop/

DAUGHTER: mucus like seaweed caught on its tongue.
    I wonder how it's still alive?/

FATHER: I'm trying my best/

DAUGHTER: each wave shakes my insides/

FATHER: I'm trying my best/

DAUGHTER: its roar rattles right fucking through me/

FATHER: don't swear/

DAUGHTER: fuck! I'm trying my best/

FATHER: to be Hard, like the floor like Facts/

DAUGHTER: it's been here before/

FATHER: like black and white Facts/

DAUGHTER: washed up on the shore/

FATHER: like Solid like Bone like Beginnings and Ends
    Like Truth/

DAUGHTER: unwanted and unwelcome.

FATHER: like Truth!

DAUGHTER: Unwelcome!

FATHER: But she is softly, softly/

DAUGHTER: praying it doesn't wake/

FATHER: softly softly/

DAUGHTER: wondering how on earth/

FATHER: softly/

DAUGHTER: spit him out onto shore/

FATHER: softly/

DAUGHTER: onto cold Fucking Floor that on a weekday
    is *spotless?!*

FATHER: And I do not not want to open my eyes and see Her eyes wide and sad looking, looking Down at me? Little ears that match her mothers/

DAUGHTER: but at the weekend?

FATHER: Her hands Softly rubbing my back. Her lips repeating the word Dad, Dad, Dad Dad Dad/

DAUGHTER: at the weekend?

FATHER: And above her nose is a crease?

DAUGHTER: Beached. And above her nose/

FATHER: is a crease?

DAUGHTER: A deep cut sliced/

FATHER: and I know I do that. Every time. Every time she has to look at me I/

DAUGHTER: you're not/

FATHER: what/

DAUGHTER: listening/

FATHER: you're not/

DAUGHTER: what/

FATHER: listening. Love?

DAUGHTER: I'm just gonna say it/

FATHER: Dad/

DAUGHTER: Dad/

FATHER: Dad, it is raining/

DAUGHTER: it is raining/

FATHER: the church it's the church/

DAUGHTER: love?/

FATHER: ringing ringing/

DAUGHTER: her Beautiful/

FATHER: but neither of us is going/

> *(The music suddenly blares loud and he thrashes violently. Rock-star air guitar, seeking oblivion. She is stood impossibly still, holding on. Sudden silence. He is startled, tries not to look it. They're both very aware of the audience and compete for our approval.)*

DAUGHTER: You're supposed to be/

FATHER: what?

DAUGHTER: The one who, who/..

FATHER: Yeah? Well sometimes, *(To us.)* sometimes things don't/

DAUGHTER: no, that's fucking bullshit/

FATHER: don't swear!

DAUGHTER: *(To us.)* You can't tell me/

FATHER: *(To us.)* there's No need/

DAUGHTER: *(To him.)* there's Every Fucking Need!

FATHER: Do you hate me?

DAUGHTER: Yes.

FATHER: .

DAUGHTER: No.

FATHER: Which?

DAUGHTER: Both.

FATHER: *(To us.)* You can't have both/

DAUGHTER: *(To us.)* I fucking can/

FATHER: *(To her.)* don't swear/

DAUGHTER: *(To him.)* Fuck Off!

    (Silence, she's surprised herself.)

FATHER: You're upset.

DAUGHTER: Yes.

FATHER: I've let you down.

DAUGHTER: Yes.

FATHER: I always let you down.

DAUGHTER: Yes.

FATHER: *(To no one and everyone.)* I've let her down.

DAUGHTER: .

FATHER: I'm sorry.

DAUGHTER: Not good enough.

FATHER: No?

DAUGHTER: No.

FATHER: Oh.

DAUGHTER: Doesn't last. Never lasts.

FATHER: Short expiry date?

(Silence, it's not funny.)

FATHER: I'm sorry.

(Silence, it's not enough.)

DAUGHTER: *(To him.)* I put the washing on.

FATHER: Thanks. Great, thanks, thank you that's/
DAUGHTER: some of your underwear was in the pile.

FATHER: Right?
DAUGHTER: Your briefs. *(To us.)* Blue. Your blue briefs.
FATHER: Yes. Well you don't actually need to/
DAUGHTER: they had shit in them.
FATHER: .
DAUGHTER: Stains. Marks. Where you'd/
FATHER: yes alright/
DAUGHTER: where you'd clearly/
FATHER: yes, thank you/
DAUGHTER: tried to wipe it/
FATHER: YES *ALRIGHT!*

(Silence, he's surprised himself.)

49

DAUGHTER: You'd shit yourself Dad. Poisoned yourself. Drank so much your body/

FATHER: yes well *embarrassing* me about it isn't/

DAUGHTER: I couldn't stop looking at it.

FATHER: .

DAUGHTER: Staring at it. The stain. And feeling so Terribly Angry at it. Which is daft really because it's not, It's fault, It's just a mark, but a very clear Visible mark an Obvious Sign that you/.. And I thought about it being in the washing machine. The water and the soap lifting it, the particles of poo lifted off the fabric and floating around, getting stuck on the other clothes in the machine maybe, or maybe they'd wash away? The germs would? I mean it's hot isn't it, it's not like a quick rinse under a tap it's. Sixty fucking degrees, or forty or, depending on, eco fucking friendly and I. I thought about the particles getting stuck to my clothes. That's possible isn't it? A possible possibility of washing my clothes with *Your Shit Stain* is that some of it could. And I'd walk around with, Your Shit, stuck on me. And I'd ingest it. I'd breathe it in, get it stuck in my lungs. I'd be breathing your shit into my lungs. Carrying particles around with me on my clothes, seeping, into my skin into the pours in my, getting into my bloodstream, into my digestive system and maybe I'd be inspired by, Infected by you and it'd make me do the same. Kick off the desire to do the same and I'd Shit my pants, Shit you out sweet Sweet release Shit you out into my knickers and leave a forever Stain.

FATHER: .

DAUGHTER: Or maybe not. Maybe I'd carry you around inside me for *years*. Like chewing gum. How long is, seven years?

50

FATHER: I'm sorry/

DAUGHTER: no.

FATHER: .

DAUGHTER: .

FATHER: I/

DAUGHTER: I chucked 'em. Couldn't risk it.

FATHER: I'm/

DAUGHTER: couldn't risk the chance/

FATHER: I/

DAUGHTER: of turning into you.

(Silence. Thick silence. He moves towards the door and she panics.)

DAUGHTER: sorry. sorry. Sorry, sorry sorry. Sorry. Sorry, sorry, sorry, sorry, Sorry, sorry sorry. Sorry, Sorry sorrysorrysorrySorrysorrysorrysorrySorrysorrysorrysorry sorrysorrysorrysorrysorrysorrysorrysorrysorrysorrysorry sorry.

(Silence, it's not enough.)

DAUGHTER: Say you Meant it Dad.

FATHER: I/..

DAUGHTER: Say you meant Every Word.

(He exits. She looks at us, waiting. He re-enters with the cassette player, returns it to its usual place. Strokes the top of it softly. They speak to us.)

DAUGHTER: I don't do that anymore/

FATHER: why? It's fun.

DAUGHTER: It's not/

FATHER: 'course it is! It's always/

DAUGHTER: hasn't been for years/

FATHER: you haven't.

DAUGHTER: Don't/

FATHER: you've forgotten how! You've lost your/

DAUGHTER: stop it/

FATHER: you look so/..

DAUGHTER: What?

FATHER: .

DAUGHTER: What/

FATHER: tight. So, Tight. You look like you Need some fun.

DAUGHTER: .

FATHER: Come dance with me.

DAUGHTER: I can't.

FATHER: Come on.

DAUGHTER: I can't.

FATHER: Come on. Have a dance/

DAUGHTER: I Can't, once I start/

FATHER: have a dance!

DAUGHTER: I can't Stop/

FATHER: come on/

DAUGHTER: and my body aches.

(He can't listen to this, is almost disgusted by it.)

DAUGHTER: And I've broken, Everything and I can't stop
and it's stopping me doing anything else and my feet are
bleeding and I desperately desperately want to but I/..

*(She stops dead and looks down at her right leg. It is dancing softly,
it has already caught the beat. She watches her leg as it builds in
confidence, enjoying the song. She looks to her dad, terrified. He
smiles. The song gets louder. They stare at each other. The song gets
louder. They dance.*

*They do the same moves, keeping eye contact, giving each other
confidence. Laughter bursts out of them as they enjoy the movement,
building in confidence and energy. Everything looks different, the
walls are suddenly more vibrant, the floor is bouncing with them,
the ceiling is raising higher, everything conspiring to give them a
good time. And the song is everywhere, filling every pour, every crack,
colouring the room and flavouring the air. They are breathing it in
and it is giving them life. Everything is growing bigger and better
by the second. They are dancing and it feels wonderful.*

*She is enjoying the dance like she's discovering her body for the first
time, falling in love with what it can do, with the movement it can
do, the shapes it can make. She expands as she explores, wanting*

more and more, she becomes powerful. He sees her power and is beyond proud, in awe of her. The song stutters and skips, he looks at the cassette player confused. It trips into a remix, something she's influencing somehow by her dance. Her power scares and delights him in almost equal measure.

The remix kicks off into something more disjointed, more fractured, more aggressive in tone. Her moves become more wild, more aggressive, more desperate. The dance for both of them becomes chaotic and animal and ugly. Spinning and spinning and spinning, lashing out, writhing and gyrating. Lights flash and the walls close in. Everything is too loud. It's chaotic, its ugly, it's frightening.

Eventually he runs out of breath and the song slows to a stop. He's grateful for the quiet, swaying in the heavy silence. She wants more, tries to dance without the music, screaming for more, for more, for more! She thrashes and thrashes. He watches her, heartbroken. She collapses. He doesn't know what to do. He softly touches her shoulder with his palm. It burns her. He sees his touch burn her and it breaks him. They curl up on the floor, the same, but separate. They breathe, and cry, or pray, or something. Lights slowly fade and we feel the bright glow of morning, of mourning, of aftermath. He looks at her. She can't look at him.)

FATHER: Sweetheart?

(She doesn't respond. He has nothing else to offer but that one word.)

*DAUGHTER: I won't stay. I/.. Be out of your hair.

FATHER: It's fine.

DAUGHTER: I just need/

FATHER: it's/

DAUGHTER: get back on my feet.

54

FATHER: Honestly, it's/..

DAUGHTER: I'm really/

FATHER: really. The least I can/..

(They look at each other. They touch their foreheads together like lions. They move apart. They exhale slowly. They agree, it's Time. She exits. He sits alone. He reaches over to his cassette player, hesitates, before hitting play. The button clicks down and we hear the first beat of the song before we cut to blackout.)

By the same author

Blush
9781786820150

Bitch Boxer
9781849434775

WWW.OBERONBOOKS.COM

Follow us on Twitter @oberonbooks
& Facebook @OberonBooksLondon